The Juicing Bible

Second Edition

Pat Crocker

Robert
ROSE

The Juicing Bible, Second Edition
Text copyright © 2000, 2008 Pat Crocker
Photographs and illustrations copyright © 2000, 2008 Robert Rose Inc.
Cover and text design copyright © 2008 Robert Rose Inc.

This is a revised and expanded edition of *The Juicing Bible*, published by Robert Ros

For complete cataloguing information, see page 366.

Disclaimer

The Juicing Bible is intended to provide information about the preparation and use of
whole foods and medicinal herbs. It is not intended as a substitute for professional m
publisher and author do not represent or warrant that the use of recipes or other infor
in this book will necessarily aid in the prevention or treatment of any disease, and spe
any liability, loss or risk, personal or otherwise, incurred as a consequence, directly or
and application of any of the contents of this book. Readers must assume sole respon
lifestyle and/or treatment program that they choose to follow. If you have questions re
of diet and health, speak to a healthcare professional.

The recipes in this book have been carefully tested by our kitchen and our tasters.
our knowledge, they are safe and nutritious for ordinary use and users. For those peop
allergies, or who have special food requirements or health issues, please read the sugg
each recipe carefully and determine whether or not they may create a problem for you
at the risk of the consumer.

We cannot be responsible for any hazards, loss or damage that may occur as a resul

For those with special needs, allergies, requirements or health problems, in the eve
please contact your medical adviser prior to the use of any recipe.

Design and Production: Joseph Gisini/PageWave Graphics Inc.
Editors: Carol Sherman and Sue Sumeraj
Proofreader: Karen Campbell-Sheviak
Indexer: Gillian Watts
Photography: Colin Erricson
Photograph of Tomato Juice Cocktail: Mark T. Shapiro
Photograph on chapter openers: istockphoto.com/arsat
Food Styling: Kathryn Robertson and Kate Bush
Prop Styling: Charlene Erricson
Illustrations: Kveta/Three In A Box

Cover image: Strawberry Sparkle, see page 204.

We acknowledge the financial support of the Government of Canada through the Boo
Development Program (BPIDP) for our publishing activities.

Published by Robert Rose Inc.
120 Eglinton Avenue East, Suite 800, Toronto, Ontario, Canada M4P 1E2
Tel: (416) 322-6552 Fax: (416) 322-6936
www.robertrose.ca

Printed and bound in Canada

11 12 13 TCP 18 17 16 15 14 13 12

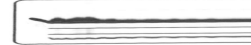